Table of Contents

Table of Contents

LifeSkills Training

Promoting Health and Personal Development

Student Guide 1

Gilbert J. Botvin, Ph.D.

Professor of Public Health and Psychiatry

Director of the Institute for Prevention Research Cornell University Medical College

Princeton Health Press
1.800.293.4969
www.lifeskillstraining.com

Botvin
LifeSkills Training

CJK 12-10

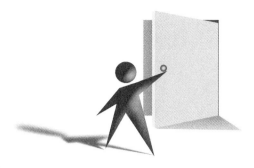

Introduction

We live in a complex and challenging world. To succeed in this world and effectively deal with the many problems facing us requires a specific set of skills. We call these skills "life skills." Surprisingly, these important skills are not usually taught to us in school; they are not usually taught to us at home, in college, or on the job. In fact, they are rarely taught at all. Instead, we are somehow expected to learn the skills we need to live happy, healthy, and successful lives totally on our own.

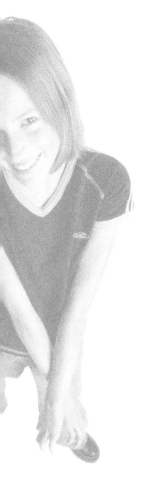

Some people do learn these "life skills" on their own, but not in any organized way. If they learn them at all, they learn them in a hit-or-miss way. Those of us who are lucky enough to learn these skills have a better chance of becoming happy, healthy, and successful. Unfortunately, most of us may go through our entire lives without learning these skills or only partially learning them.

The Purpose of This Program

The *LifeSkills Training* program was developed by Dr. Gilbert J. Botvin, a psychologist at Cornell University, to provide an organized way for all junior high school students to learn these important skills. Dr. Botvin discovered that students who received this program not only were better prepared to deal with the challenges of life, but were less likely to smoke, drink, or use drugs. The *LifeSkills Training* program is an exciting new breakthrough which not only prevents tobacco, alcohol and drug abuse, but teaches the knowledge and skills necessary to:

- Increase your self-esteem
- Increase your ability to make decisions and solve problems
- Communicate effectively
- Avoid misunderstandings
- Manage anxiety
- Make new friends
- Stand up for your rights
- Say "no" to unfair requests
- Resist advertising pressures
- Resist pressure to use drugs

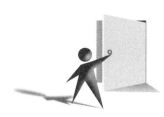

Introduction

Your Student Guide

The **Student Guide** was developed to help the students taking part in the *LifeSkills Training* program. This guide contains information taught in the program and provides step-by-step instructions on how to use the "life skills" taught in the program. The **Student Guide** is an important source of information which can be referred to over and over again until you've mastered the skills taught in the program or to review any of these skills from time-to-time in the future.

Class Material and Practice

Most of the material contained in the **Student Guide** will be covered in class by your teacher. The **Student Guide** includes material that your teacher will refer to in class, some general background information, and exercises to be completed at home or in class. These exercises are designed to help you get the most out of the *LifeSkills Training* program; therefore, it is important for you to do them. In addition to filling out the exercises in your **Student Guide,** it is important for you to practice the skills taught in the program. It is only by practicing these skills and applying them to your life every day that you will fully master them.

Self-Improvement Project

An important part of the *LifeSkills Training* program is a self-improvement project. This project is valuable because it teaches you how to identify things about yourself that you would like to change, set goals, and then progress forward step-by-step until you have succeeded in changing yourself or learning a particular skill. Forms are included in the **Student Guide** for you to set goals and keep track of your progress as you work toward those goals.

How the Program Is Organized

After a general introduction by your teacher, the program starts with information and skills that will help you develop a positive self-image. Next, the program focuses on learning how to make decisions without being influenced too much by other people, by advertisements, and by things you see or hear in the media (TV, Internet, newspapers, magazines, etc.). The program also includes material on how to resist pressures to smoke, drink, or use other drugs. The program then focuses on the best ways of dealing with anxiety, communicating with others, and building friendships. It ends by teaching skills for saying "no" to unfair requests or offers to use drugs. This is a great program which has already been helpful to thousands of students just like you. We are confident that you will find it to be personally valuable and fun. Above right are the rules to be followed in the classroom:

Ground Rules

• Everyone sits in a circle.

• Only one person talks at a time.

• No one should be forced to participate if he/she really does not want to, although everyone is encouraged to do so.

• Students are free to express their opinions or participate in group activities without being subjected to criticism.

• Anything discussed in the group remains confidential.

In the space below, list additional rules suggested by the class:

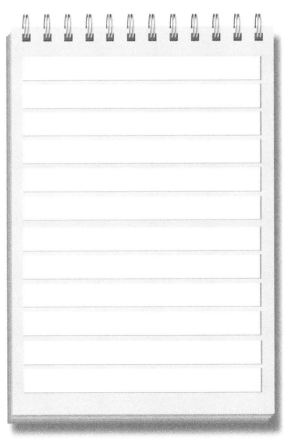

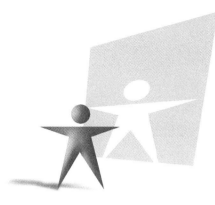

Self-Image

and

Self-Improvement

Self-Image and How It Develops

What do we mean by the term self-image? Self-image is simply how we see ourselves; the mental picture or image we have of ourselves. The way we see ourselves is formed largely by our past experiences (successes and failures) and what people have told us about ourselves. If all your teachers told you that you were smart, you would probably think you were smart! If people told you that you were good at sports and you did well at sports, you would in all likelihood think of yourself as a good athlete. Self-image is generally a reflection of who we really are. However, people don't always see themselves as they really are.

How Self-Image Affects Behavior

Why does it matter if we see ourselves accurately? It's important for two reasons. First, how we see ourselves is important because it affects how we behave, what we do, and how well we do it. It affects how hard we try. For example, people who think they are good math students will work hard and usually will get good grades in math. People tend to act like the person they think they are.

A second reason that self-image is important is that it affects how good you feel about yourself. People who feel good about themselves are more confident, more satisfied, more successful, do better in school, and are more popular than people who see themselves in a negative light. People who have a positive self-image are also less likely to smoke, drink, use drugs, or engage in other unhealthy activities.

Improving Your Self and Your Self-Image

Although most of us have a general self-image, it is usually made up of a number of separate self-images relating to ourselves in specific situations. For example, one person may be a good baseball player, a bad swimmer, a good writer, an average math student, etc., all at the same time.

You can do several things to improve your self-image and self-esteem. First, never form a negative image of yourself after one or two bad experiences. Second, take stock. Look at yourself as realistically as possible. Identify your strengths and weaknesses. Third, work on improving in areas where you are weak. You can develop a more positive self-image by setting and achieving goals, by deciding what you'd like to change about yourself or what you'd like to accomplish, and then doing it.

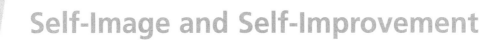

Self-Image and Self-Improvement

Describe yourself as you are now and as you would like to be, using three adjectives or short phrases.

How I See Myself

Myself Now

With Friends

Myself Now	Myself As I Would Like To Be
1. mean	fun to be around
2. selfish	funny
3. probably annoying	happy

At School

1. a good worker	a good worker
2. independent	independent
3. quiet	quiet

At Home

1. bored	funny
2. nice	nice
3. quiet	fun to be around

In General

1. a good person	a good person
2. sensative	sensative
3. fun to be around	funny

I am; Competitive, overwhelming, and annoying.

In the space to the right list your strengths and weaknesses.

List five things about yourself that you would like to change or improve. Rate how important it is to you to change each of these five things.

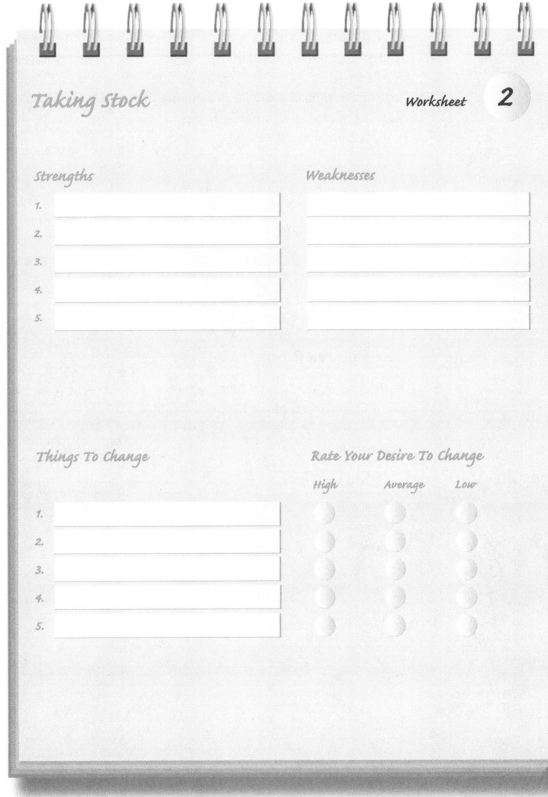

Taking Stock

Strengths

1.
2.
3.
4.
5.

Weaknesses

1.
2.
3.
4.
5.

Things To Change

1.
2.
3.
4.
5.

Rate Your Desire To Change

High	Average	Low

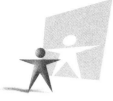

Self-Image and Self-Improvement

Setting and Achieving Personal Goals

How to Set Goals

1. Pick a goal that is realistic. Set a goal for yourself which is possible for you to accomplish within a reasonable amount of time (for example, by the end of the school semester).

2. Pick a goal that is manageable, that you can break down into a series of small steps (or sub-goals). The best way to change a behavior is to do it in small steps.

3. Pick a goal which is measurable (for example, how far you jog) so you can tell whether you have achieved it or how much further you have to improve before you do.

4. Pick something that is meaningful to you, something that you really want to do rather than something you feel you should do.

Tips for Achieving Your Goals

1. Have a positive attitude. Believe in yourself and your ability to reach the goal that you set for yourself.

2. Don't be afraid to make mistakes. It's all part of learning and making progress toward your goal.

3. If you don't reach a particular goal or sub-goal, don't think of it as a failure. Think of it as a learning experience, as a step toward achieving your goal. Identify what went wrong and correct it.

4. Praise yourself for any progress that you make toward achieving your goal. Tell your friends or parents, and reward yourself.

5. Identify any areas that need further improvement and work on them with confidence and determination.

6. Use your imagination. Spend some time each day "seeing" yourself achieving your goal.

Pick a goal from the ones you listed on **Worksheet 2, Taking Stock.** Write it in the space provided to the right along with a series of smaller sub-goals leading to it and the date you expect to reach it. (You should generally allow about a week for reaching each sub-goal.) Put a check mark next to the "Yes" or "No" to show whether you achieved each of the sub-goals.

Recording My Progress

Goal:

Date	Sub-goal	Achieved Sub-goal	
		Yes	No
		○	○
		○	○
		○	○
		○	○
		○	○
		○	○
		○	○
		○	○
		○	○
		○	○
		○	○
		○	○

Making
Decisions

Deciding Things On Your Own

As you get older, you will need to make more and more decisions on your own. Some of these may be very difficult. To make the best possible decisions, you will need to be aware of the people or things around you that can influence your decisions (such as your parents, friends, TV, movies, and advertisements). You will also need to learn an organized method for making decisions. Being aware of the factors that might influence your decisions and knowing how to make decisions will help you to make the best possible decisions for you.

A Simple Method for Making Better Decisions

Most people make all their decisions in the same way, without realizing the difference between simple choices, everyday decisions, and major decisions. Simple choices (whether to eat vanilla or chocolate ice cream) can be decided based on what you like. Other decisions should be made after carefully thinking about the possible consequences or outcomes of different decisions. To do this as well as possible and make the best decisions, you should learn to use the 3-Step method described here.

The 3 Cs of Effective Decision-Making

Step 1: **Clarify** the decision to be made (what is the decision that you need to make).

Step 2: **Consider** the possible alternatives (think about the different things you might decide to do) and the consequences of choosing each alternative; collect any additional information needed. (If you are trying to solve a problem, think up as many solutions as possible).

Step 3: **Choose** the best alternative and take the necessary action. Be sure to follow through on your decision.

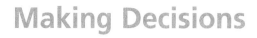

Making Decisions

Make a list of the most important decisions you have to make everyday or almost everyday at home, school, or with friends. Indicate with a check mark whether you make those decisions **On Your Own** or whether you are influenced by **Parents, Friends, Teachers,** or the **Media (TV, movies, magazines, newspapers, DVDs, books, etc.).** If you are influenced by more than one, check as many sources of influence as apply to each decision.

Everyday Decisions   **Worksheet** 4

Decisions

At Home	On My Own	Parents	Friends	Teachers	Media
1.	○	○	○	○	○
2.	○	○	○	○	○
3.	○	○	○	○	○
4.	○	○	○	○	○
5.	○	○	○	○	○

At School	On My Own	Parents	Friends	Teachers	Media
1.	○	○	○	○	○
2.	○	○	○	○	○
3.	○	○	○	○	○
4.	○	○	○	○	○
5.	○	○	○	○	○

With Friends	On My Own	Parents	Friends	Teachers	Media
1.	○	○	○	○	○
2.	○	○	○	○	○
3.	○	○	○	○	○
4.	○	○	○	○	○
5.	○	○	○	○	○

*Read each of the situations described to the right and (1) **clarify** (identify) the problem, (2) list and then **consider** the possible solutions (choices) and their likely consequences, and (3) **choose** the best solution.*

Situation: Your teacher gave your class a homework assignment that is due the next day and will help determine the grade you get in the course. That night is an important basketball game that all of your friends will be attending. If you go to the basketball game, you won't have time to do your homework, but you know someone who might let you copy her homework.

Problem:

Possible Solution	Possible Consequences
1.	
2.	
3.	

My Decision:

Situation: Your friends want to get together at your house after school when no one is home and drink beer. You really want to be with your friends and have fun, but you know your parents will be mad if you do and you'll get in a lot of trouble.

Problem:

Possible Solutions	Possible Consequences
1.	
2.	
3.	

My Decision:

Making Decisions

Pick two decisions that you have to make now or sometime in the near future. Briefly describe the situation and then (1) **clarify** (identify) the decision to be made or problem to be solved, (2) list and then **consider** the possible solutions (choices) and their likely consequences, and (3) **choose** the best alternative.

My Decision Making Planner

Worksheet **6**

Describe the Situation:

Problem:

Possible Solutions

1.
2.
3.

Possible Consequences

My Decision:

Describe the Situation:

Problem

Possible Solutions

1.
2.
3.

Possible Consequences

My Decision:

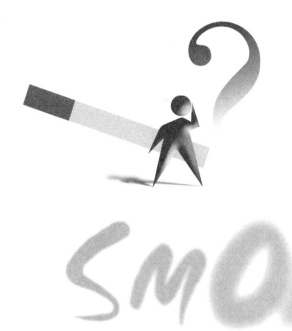

Myths and

Realities

Smoking: Myths and Realities

Myth: Cigarette smoking is not as dangerous as some people say.

Reality: Most health experts agree that cigarette smoking is one of the most serious causes of death and disability in this country.

Myth: It's easy to quit smoking.

Reality: Most people are unsuccessful at quitting smoking, even though 1/2 of all smokers have tried to quit at least once.

Myth: Smoking is not something I will have to worry about until I'm old.

Reality: Smoking is something that hurts you now. It hurts you physically by decreasing your ability to perform strenuous activities, elevating carbon monoxide levels and decreasing endurance, staining teeth and fingers, affecting your sense of taste, causing you to smell like smoke, and costing over $1,000 a year.

Myth: Most people smoke cigarettes.

Reality: Relatively few people smoke cigarettes and even fewer are likely to smoke in the future.

Myth: Smoking is cool and sophisticated.

Reality: Smoking has become socially unacceptable in most places.

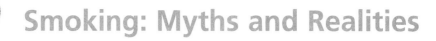

Smoking: Myths and Realities

Write down the class estimates of the percentage of teenagers who smoke, drink, and use marijuana and other drugs at least once a month. Compare these estimates to recent results of a national survey of 8th, 10th, and 12th graders by The National Institute on Drug Abuse.

Who's Using Drugs?

Worksheet **7**

Substance	Class Estimate	8th Grade	10th Grade	12th Grade
Cigarettes		6.5	13.1	20.1
Smokeless Tobacco		3.7	6.5	8.4
Alcohol		14.9	30.4	43.5
Marijuana/Hashish		6.5	15.9	20.6
Inhalants		3.8	2.2	1.2
Cocaine		0.8	0.9	1.3
Crack		0.5	0.4	0.6
Methamphetamine		0.5	0.6	0.5
Tranquilizers		1.2	2.0	2.7
Hallucinogens		0.9	1.4	1.6
LSD		0.5	0.5	0.5
Heroin		0.4	0.4	0.4
Steroids		0.4	0.5	1.0

Source: Johnston, L.D., O'Malley, P.M., Bachman, J.G. & Schulenberg, J.E. (December 14, 2009). "Teen marijuana use tilts up, while some drugs decline in use." University of Michigan News Service: Ann Arbor, MI. Retrieved 12/02/2010 from http://www.monitoringthefuture.org

Smoking and Your Body

5.00
x   7
$35.00   weekly

5.00
30
$150.00   Monthly

365
5.00
$1,875.00   yearly

Parts of the Body Affected

Ears
- Affects the nerves and blood vessels in the ears and may lead to hearing loss.

Eyes
- Causes the eyes to become red and may lead to loss of eyesight.

Mouth
- Harms the skin covering the lips, tongue, and throat, and may cause food to taste funny.

- Causes bad coughs.

- Causes bad breath and mouth infections.

Nose
- Decreases your ability to smell.

Skin
- Causes the temperature of the skin to drop.

- Causes wrinkles on the face to appear quickly.

Lungs
- Makes it harder to breathe normally which makes it harder for you to do well in sports.

Heart
- Closes off blood vessels making the heart work harder to pump blood through them.

Other Ways Smoking Can Hurt You

You probably already know that smoking causes heart disease, cancer, emphysema, and strokes. But did you also know that smoking gives you bad breath, makes your clothes smell, and stains your teeth? Who wants to be friends with someone like that!

Smoking is Not Popular

Before anyone knew how bad smoking was, many people smoked. Some people even thought it was cool. But that's not true today. Smoking is a thing of the past. It's not cool to smoke these days. The only people who smoke are people who are too hooked to quit.

Recent surveys indicate that only about 3% of eighth graders, 6% of tenth graders and 11% of twelfth graders smoke cigarettes everyday. Only about 20% of adults smoke regularly. This means that most people in the United States do not smoke cigarettes.

Non-Smokers' Rights

People who don't smoke are becoming more assertive regarding their right to breathe clean air and more vocal in their objections to smoking. The main reason non-smokers have begun standing up for their rights is the growing scientific evidence that sidestream smoke (smoke from the lighted tip of a cigarette between puffs) has a higher concentration of some of the hazardous substances than does mainstream smoke (smoke inhaled by the smoker). Non-smokers who are in a room with smokers are forced to breathe in these substances and to become involuntary smokers. Involuntary smoking is dangerous, according to the results of recent scientific studies, increasing nonsmokers' risk of getting smoking-related diseases.

List your personal reasons for not wanting to become a cigarette smoker in the space provided to the right.

My Reasons For Not Smoking

1.

2.

3.

4.

5.

6.

7.

8.

9.

10.

smokin

and

Biofeedback

60-90

Immediate Effects of Cigarette Smoking

Smoking Can Affect You Now

Many of the reasons doctors and other health experts give for not smoking have to do with the fact that smoking causes a number of diseases such as heart disease and cancer. These diseases take a long time to develop. Some of these diseases may take as much as 20 or 30 years to develop.

Because it takes so long to experience the symptoms of these diseases, smoking may not seem that bad. In fact, some teenagers may not even believe that smoking will hurt them. They think that adults just talk about the dangers of smoking to scare them. The problem is, even though it may not seem like smoking is hurting your body, by the time you get a disease caused by smoking, it is usually too late.

What many people don't realize is that smoking does have an effect on your body, and that effect is immediate. It occurs within seconds, and can be measured in several different ways. Some of the things that happen after you smoke a cigarette are as follows: your heart beats faster, your hand steadiness decreases, the amount of carbon monoxide in your lungs increases, the temperature of your skin goes down, and the pattern of your brain waves changes.

Heart Rate and Smoking

Heart rate is the number of times that your heart beats each minute. Most people have a heart rate between 60 and 90 beats per minute. Most smokers have faster heart rates than non-smokers.

Smoking and Biofeedback

Why Smoking Makes Your Heart Beat Faster

Nicotine (another chemical in cigarettes) increases the heart rate by acting on a part of the body called the adrenal glands, found in the kidneys, causing them to release powerful chemicals into the body. These cause the walls of the heart to contract harder and more often.

Because nicotine causes an increase in the heart's activity, the heart needs more oxygen. At the same time, carbon monoxide that is inhaled by the smoker from the cigarette pushes out the oxygen in the blood, forcing the heart to work harder to get more oxygen to the body.

Physical activity also causes the body to need more oxygen, so that the heart beats faster. This means that cigarette smoking places an extra strain on the heart beyond its normal work. Over time, this may cause such severe damage to the heart that it could stop working. We call this a heart attack.

Interesting Facts

• People who don't smoke and who exercise regularly (for example, marathon runners) may sometimes have a normal resting heart rate as low as 30–40 beats per minute.

• Cigarette smoking decreases the delivery of oxygen to the muscles during vigorous exercise, making the effort of the activity more difficult than usual.

• Nicotine increases levels of blood lactate. When exercising, elevated levels of blood lactate can make people feel fatigued or feel like quitting.

• In some people, cigarette smoke can trigger asthma symptoms, making it nearly impossible to exercise until the symptoms subside.

Things to Remember

- The speed at which your heart beats changes throughout the day. Several things can affect how fast or slow your heart beats. They include physical exercise, emotions, relaxation, and cigarette smoking.

- Smokers have higher heart rates due to the carbon monoxide and nicotine in cigarette smoke.

- People who smoke have a greater risk of heart disease and heart attacks.

Hand-Steadiness

Another effect cigarette smoking has on your body is that it decreases hand-steadiness. In other words, it causes your hand to shake more. Although this is not always so bad that you can see it, it can be measured using what is called a hand-steadiness or tremor-tension test. It is the nicotine in the cigarette smoke that makes this happen. Nicotine is a stimulant which speeds up your heart and the rate at which you breathe. Most smokers believe that smoking "calms them down," but it really does the opposite.

Things to Remember

- Smoking decreases hand-steadiness.

- The nicotine in cigarette smoke acts as a stimulant.

- Rather than "calming you down," smoking makes you more nervous.

How to Take Someone's Pulse

Before you can do this experiment, you must know how to take someone's pulse. Place your first and second fingers of your right hand on the inside of the right wrist of a smoker. The picture below shows you how to do this. Next, count the number of thumps (pulsations) that you feel. Use a watch with a second hand, so that you can count the number of pulsations you feel in one minute. This number (pulsations in one minute) is called the pulse rate.

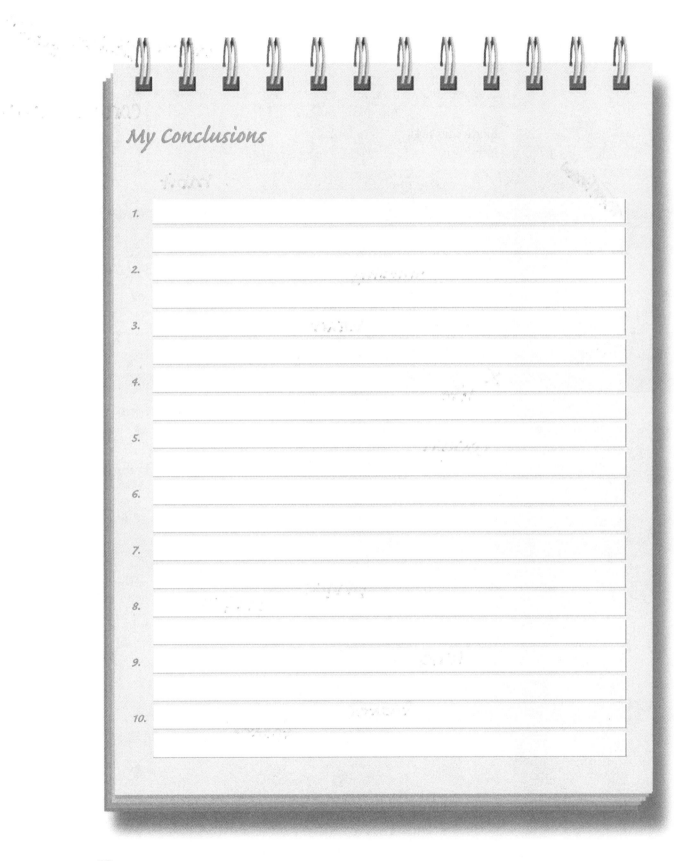

My Conclusions

1.

2.

3.

4.

5.

6.

7.

8.

9.

10.

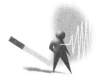

Smoking and Biofeedback

Puzzle Clues

1. If you smoke for a long time, _____ builds up in your lungs and makes them look black. (3 letters)

2. The cigarette brand which advertises a macho image and outdoor living is called _____. (8 letters)

3. Everybody knows that cigarette smoking is *on healthy*. (9 letters)

4. Smoking cigarettes increases your chances of having a *hEArt* attack. (5 letters)

5. Cigarette smoking shortens your *life*. (4 letters)

6. You may develop a hacking *cough* if you smoke. (5 letters)

7. The nicotine in cigarettes is a known _____. (6 letters)

8. One reason not to smoke is that you will develop yellow *plaque* on your teeth and fingers. (6 letters) *plaque*

9. Cigarette smoking is a major cause of *lung* cancer. (4 letters)

10. Smoking cigarettes makes your heart beat *faster*. (6 letters) *faster*

carbon ~~*dioxide*~~ *monoxide*

11. The colorless and odorless gas in cigarette smoke is called _____. (14 letters) *Carbon monoxide*

12. People who smoke cigarettes every day find that smoking is a difficult *habit* to break. (5 letters) *habit*

13. Smoking cigarettes has become less socially _____ as more and more adults are giving up smoking. (10 letters)

14. Scientists have discovered that sidestream _____ is potentially dangerous to the nonsmoker. (5 letters)

15. _____ teenagers are non-smokers. (4 letters)

16. Carbon monoxide forces out the oxygen from the body's _____ blood cells. (3 letters)

Unhealthy

Smoking Word Puzzle

Directions: Hidden in this puzzle are words that have to do with some of the things you have learned about cigarette smoking during the LifeSkills Training Program. These words are written forward, backward, and diagonally throughout the puzzle. To the left are some clues to help you find these words. Circle the words after you find them.

```
z  v  t  o  l  k  f  s  n  i  a  t  s  r
q  w  i  n  u  c  c  m  n  x  f  y  e  m
o  v  b  r  n  f  j  o  m  n  p  h  l  a
r  r  a  o  g  t  s  k  j  e  j  t  b  k
o  p  h  d  r  i  d  e  g  r  i  l  a  r
b  p  k  a  o  f  n  s  b  v  c  a  t  f
l  d  e  p  h  r  c  i  f  o  b  e  p  j
r  h  y  u  b  i  v  d  a  u  j  h  e  a
a  h  u  n  v  e  z  d  s  s  i  n  c  l
m  g  n  w  y  n  i  o  t  z  l  u  c  z
   u  y  o  t  d  j  x  e  s  y  i  a  o
   o  c  r  v  s  q  s  r  a  t  t  m  m
f  c  e  g  s  b  o  c  l  r  c  a  c  s
   d  i  x  o  n  o  m  n  o  b  r  a  c
```

35

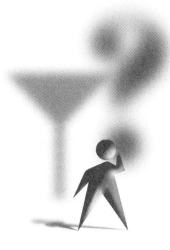

Alcohol

Myths and Realities

Drinking Fact Sheet

What is Alcohol

Alcohol is a drug contained in beverages (drinks) such as beer, wine, wine coolers, or liquor. After you drink it, alcohol is absorbed through the walls of the stomach and intestines, directly into the bloodstream. Then, it travels through the blood to the brain. Once it reaches the brain, it depresses or slows down the brain's activity.

What Alcohol Does

A Small Amount of Alcohol

• Slows down the ability to think clearly and make decisions

• Causes people to feel more daring than usual and take risks

A Larger Amount of Alcohol

• Slows down other areas of the brain and nervous system

• Causes dizziness

• Decreases coordination

• Decreases reaction time

• Makes it harder to speak, walk, and stay awake

• Causes some people to pass out

How Alcohol Affects Behavior

In addition to these effects, drinking alcohol also can lead to fighting, arguing, and violence; talking louder than usual; silliness, giddiness, and giggling; and other foolish or obnoxious behavior.

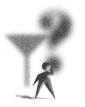

Alcohol: Myths and Realities

Reasons Why Many People Don't Drink

Many people do not drink or, if they do, they drink only once in awhile. Here are some of the reasons people give for not drinking:

- Don't like the taste.

- Don't like getting drunk.

- Don't want to get fat.

- It's against their family values.

- It's against their religious values.

- It's illegal.

- Need to stay in shape for sports.

- Don't want to look stupid.

- Don't want to look foolish.

- Drinking isn't cool.

- Want to stay in control.

- Want to think clearly.

Getting a Grip On Reality

Myth: The best way to get "high" is to drink or take drugs.

Reality: Alcohol and drugs produce a temporary "high". With alcohol, the "high" or good feeling it produces goes away after it wears off. This "up" period is followed by a "down" period where people generally feel tired, depressed, and anxious. The best way to get "high" is the natural way. Some of the ways of achieving a natural "high" are through exercise, sports, dance, music, art, achievement, prayer, meditation, friendship, and love, just to name a few.

Myth: It takes a real tough guy or girl to hold a lot of alcohol.

Reality: Like other drugs, the more alcohol someone drinks the more it takes to cause the same effects. This is because people's bodies gradually become tolerant to alcohol. An important point to keep in mind is that as tolerance increases so does a person's physical dependence on alcohol.

Myth: My friends will think I'm a wimp if I don't drink a lot.

Reality: Here's a secret: most people don't really notice how much others are drinking or even what they are drinking.

Myth: It's OK to just drink beer or wine.

Reality: A can of beer or 8 ounces of wine contains about 1 ounce of alcohol.

Myth: Drinking alcohol helps people to sleep better.

Reality: If you drink enough alcohol it can cause you to go to sleep. However, like all depressant drugs, it does not put you into a restful and relaxing state of sleep. The kind of sleep produced by alcohol is not the same as normal sleep. You will tend to wake up feeling tired, grouchy, and nervous.

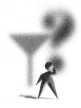

Alcohol: Myths and Realities

List your own personal reasons for not drinking alcoholic beverages such as wine, beer, or hard liquor in the space to the right.

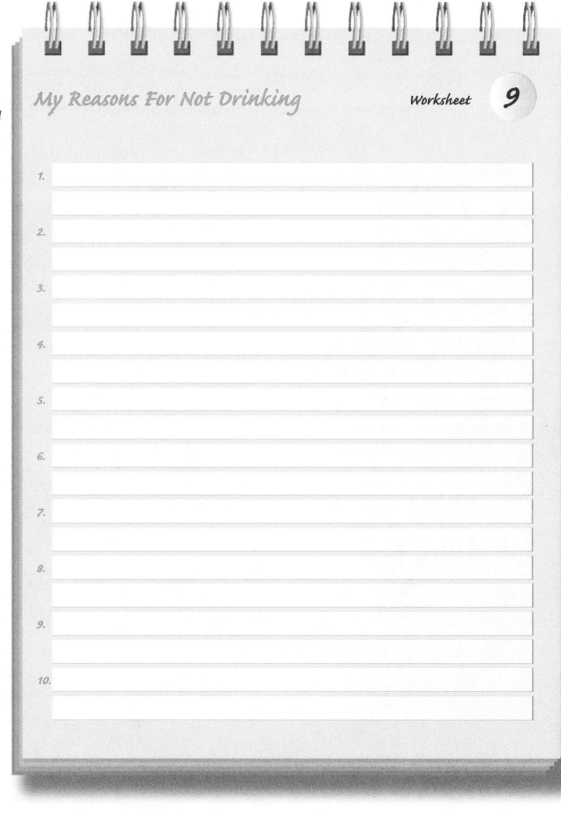

My Reasons For Not Drinking

1.

2.

3.

4.

5.

6.

7.

8.

9.

10.

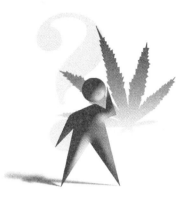

What is Marijuana

Marijuana is a dried mixture of leaves, vines, seeds, and stems of a hemp plant called cannabis sativa. It is generally used to make homemade cigarettes called "joints" or "reefers" and smoked.

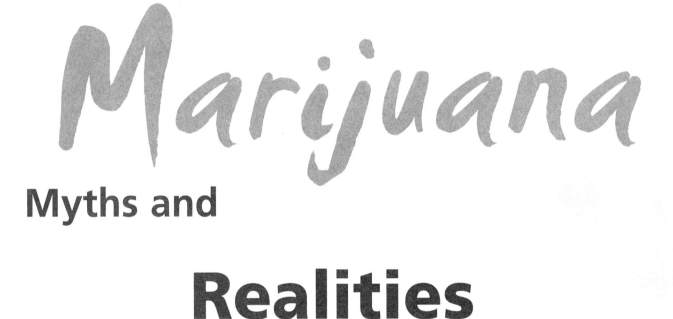

Marijuana
Myths and
Realities

What Does Marijuana Do

Marijuana affects the person smoking it within minutes. Marijuana produces a "high" or state of intoxication similar to alcohol. However, getting "high" is not the only thing marijuana does to people who smoke it. Here is a list of the things marijuana can do to people who smoke it. Scientists have discovered that marijuana:

- Causes the heart to beat faster and work harder.

- Raises some people's blood pressure.

- Makes your hands less steady.

- Causes people to feel sleepy.

- Makes it unsafe to drive a car or operate machines.

- Makes it harder to pay attention.

- Makes it harder to learn new things.

- Makes it harder to remember things.

- Makes some people feel nervous and confused.

- Makes some people feel depressed.

Most of these things go away after the marijuana wears off—which is usually in about 3 hours.

Can Marijuana Do Any Permanent Damage to the Body

Some of the things marijuana does can be permanent. Since marijuana smoke contains carbon monoxide and tar, it causes some of the same kinds of problems as smoking cigarettes. For example, it can affect people's breathing. And scientists think that, like cigarettes, smoking marijuana regularly for many years may cause certain types of cancer.

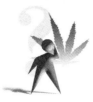

Marijuana: Myths and Realities

List your own personal reasons for not using marijuana.

My Reasons For Not Smoking Marijuana

1.

2.

3.

4.

5.

6.

7.

8.

9.

10.

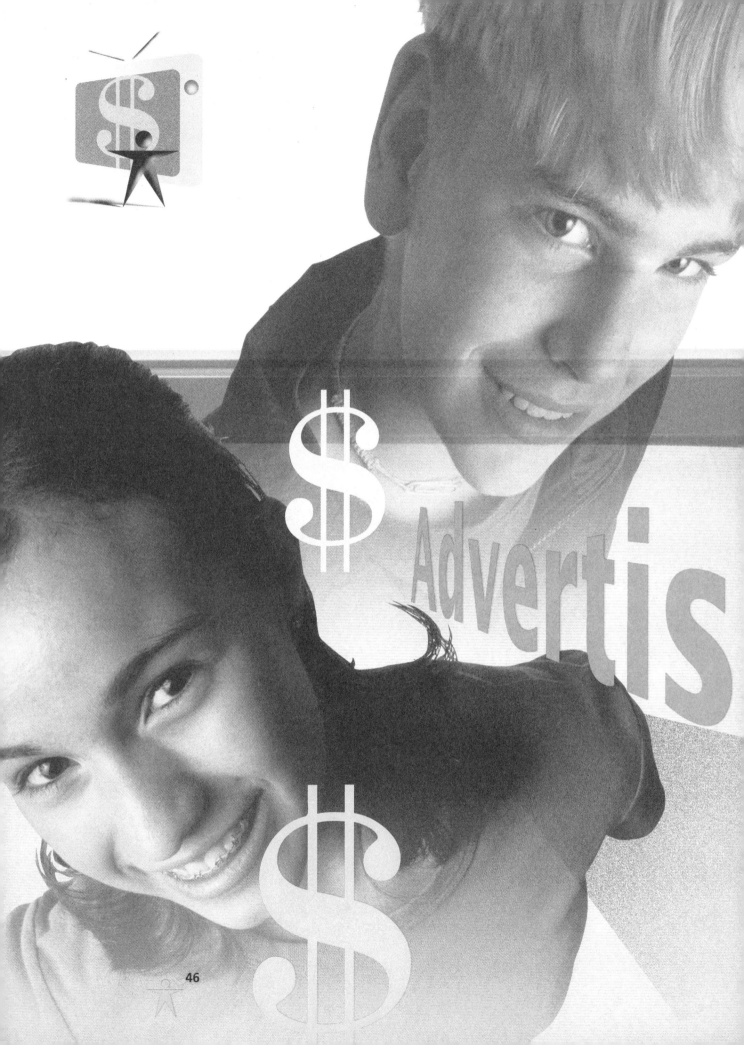

Common Advertising Techniques

One of the most powerful sources of influence on the decisions we make as consumers comes from advertisements (ads) designed to get us to buy a particular product or service. Advertisers "target" a particular group of people (e.g., parents, teenagers) who are likely to buy the product being advertised. They also use special methods or techniques to sell their products that they think will work well for a particular type of product and target group. The techniques used by advertisers usually include both a stated message (what the ad actually says) and an implied or hidden message (what is implied by either the stated message or the overall "look" or "sound" of an ad).

Some common advertising methods or techniques are listed on the next page. If you realize that advertising is intended to get you to buy a product and learn to identify common advertising techniques, you will be better able to make the decisions you want instead of being influenced by ads to make decisions that advertisers want you to make.

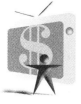

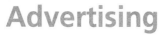

Advertising

Celebrity Endorsement: Has famous or well-known people (for example, movie stars or athletes) talk about how great the product is or even that they use it themselves. Creates the impression that the product must be good if they use it, and if you want to be like them you should use it too.

Voice of Authority: Has experts or authorities such as doctors or scientists (or actors playing the part of experts) talk about the effectiveness of products such as tooth paste or pain medicine. Since they are experts, advertisers count on the fact that consumers are likely to believe what they say about how well the product works.

Scientific Evidence: Presents "facts" and statistics from surveys supporting the effectiveness of particular products. This is often combined with the Voice of Authority technique in an effort to make the ad even more convincing.

Comparisons Tests and Opinion Polls: Presents the results of consumer opinion polls or "taste tests" involving direct comparisons of similar (competing) products. These ads are intended to show that more people like brand A than brand B, or that product X is stronger, safer, lighter, less expensive, etc. than other similar products.

Demonstrations: Intended to show how well a product works (usually under the most favorable conditions possible). Some of these demonstrations have been found to be rigged by advertisers to make the product look much better than it really is. Frequently used for household products (such as dishwashing soap, window cleaners, floor cleaners, stain-removers, dishwashers, vacuum cleaners, glue, etc.).

Bandwagon Appeal: Intended to create the impression that everybody is using a particular product and because everybody is using it you should too.

Romance/Sex Appeal: Uses very attractive models in a way that implies that using the product will make the person using it more romantically or sexually attractive.

Maturity/Sophistication Appeal: Intended to show that if you buy a certain product you will be more grown-up, sophisticated, and fashionable.

Fun/Relaxation Appeal: Intended to sell a product by convincing you that it will help you to have more fun or feel more relaxed.

Popularity Appeal: Intended to convince you to buy a certain product by implying that if you use it you will be more popular.

The "Deal" Appeal: Tries to create a sense of urgency and excitement by implying that this is a deal that is too good to pass up. Generally focuses on price and creates a sense of urgency by saying that the deal will end soon because the sale price is only good for a few days and/or there is only a limited supply of the product.

Advertising

Write the names of two general products or services being advertised, a brief description of the ad, the target group, the stated message(s), the implied or hidden message(s), and the ad technique(s) used to sell these products.

Practice Analyzing Ads

Worksheet **11**

Product Name

Brief Description of Advertisement

Target Group

Stated Message(s)

Implied Message(s)

Technique(s) Used

Write the name of a tobacco and alcohol product being advertised, a brief description of the ad, the target group, the stated message(s), the implied or hidden message(s), and the ad technique(s) used to sell these products.

Practice Analyzing Tobacco and Alcohol Ads

Tobacco Ad

Product Name

Brief Description of Advertisement

Target Group

Stated Messages

Implied Message(s)

Technique(s) Used

Alcohol Ad

51

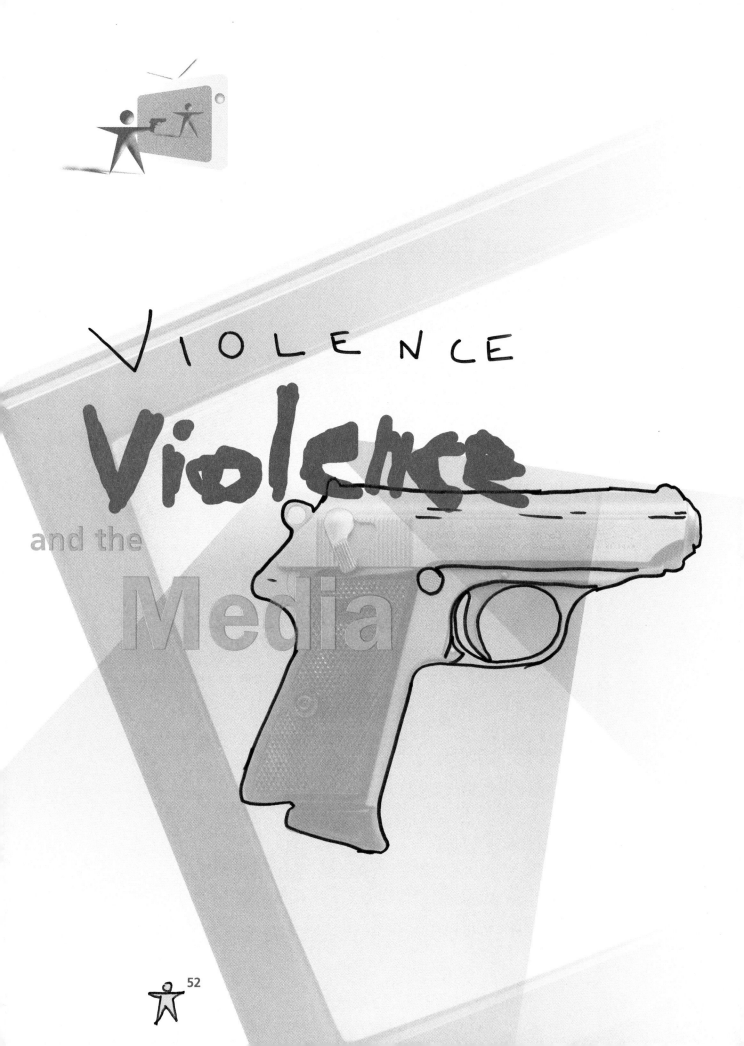

VIOLENCE

Violence

and the Media

List the TV shows and movies you watch for a week. Check whether the main characters in each show smoke, drink, use drugs, or act violently.

Name of Movie or Show	Smoke	Drink	Drug	Violence
FAMILY GUY	✓	✓	✓	✓
SOUTH PARK		✓	✓	✓
HAPPY GILMORE	✓	✓		✓
TOSH.O	✓	✓	✓	✓
GRAND THEFT AUTO	✓	✓	✓	✓
CALL OF DUTY				✓

Choose one or two violent shows. Count the number of violent acts in each one. (A violent act is an act or threat that hurts a person or object physically, such as hitting, kicking, and shooting, or verbally, such as screaming and shouting.)

Name of Show

Description of Act

1.
2.
3.
4.
5.

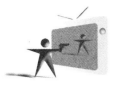

Violence and the Media

Watching TV (Continued)

Name of Show

Description of Act

1.

2.

3.

4.

5.

Take a reality check when you watch your favorite movies or TV shows. Questions to ask:

Reality Checks

1. Is this what happens in real life?

2. Do I agree with this image?

3. Is there a good reason for this violence?

   Is it trying to make a point, or is it just there to give viewers a safe thrill?

4. What would be the consequences of this violence in real life?

   Are these consequences shown?

5. Are the good guys always right no matter what they do?

6. Are the bad guys shown as deserving what they get, even if it's vigilante, or illegal violence?

7. Is this the best way to resolve this conflict?

8. How else might this conflict be resolved?

Coping
with
Anxiety

How to Decrease Your Anxiety

Relaxation Exercise

1. Sit quietly in a comfortable position.

2. Close your eyes.

3. Slowly relax all of the muscles in your body beginning with your toes, working your way up the rest of your body to the muscles in your neck and head.

4. After you've relaxed all the muscles in your body, imagine yourself in a peaceful and relaxing place (for example, lying on a beach). Whatever place you choose, think of yourself completely relaxed and without a care in the world.

5. Imagine yourself in this place as clearly as possible.

6. Practice this exercise as often as possible, at least once a day for about ten minutes each time.

Mental Rehearsal

1. Imagine yourself in an important situation (for example, asking someone out for a date) feeling completely relaxed and confident.

2. Mentally practice what you will say and/or do and how you will deal with all the possible things that might happen.

3. Do this over and over again until you begin to feel more relaxed and confident.

Deep Breathing

1. Breathe in deeply from your diaphragm for a count of 4.

2. Hold it for a count of 4.

3. Breathe out for a count of 4.

4. Repeat 4 or 5 times.

Coping With Anxiety

Describe two situations which make you feel very anxious and check off the signs of anxiety that you experienced.

Dealing With Anxiety: Situations Making Me Feel Anxious

Situation 1

Anxiety Signs (Check off those you felt in the situation above.)

- ◯ "Butterflies" in the stomach
- ◯ Rapid heart beat
- ◯ Shaky voice
- ◯ Muscle Tension

- ◯ Sweating hands
- ◯ Dry mouth
- ◯ Difficulty holding hands still
- ◯ Difficulty concentrating

Situation 2

Anxiety Signs

- ◯ "Butterflies" in the stomach
- ◯ Rapid heart beat
- ◯ Shaky voice
- ◯ Muscle Tension

- ◯ Sweating hands
- ◯ Dry Mouth
- ◯ Difficulty holding hands still
- ◯ Difficulty concentrating

Rate how anxious (nervous) you usually feel in each situation listed to the right.

Rating How Anxious You Feel

Situation

	High	Average	Low
Taking a test	○	○	○
Giving a report in front of the class	○	○	○
Making a speech in front of a group	○	○	○
Meeting New People	○	○	○
Starting a conversation with someone you just met	○	○	○
Giving someone a compliment	○	○	○
Telling someone that you like them	○	○	○
Asking someone out on a date	○	○	○
Asking someone for a favor	○	○	○
Competing in sports	○	○	○
Singing or playing a musical instrument in front of a group	○	○	○
Making an important decision	○	○	○
Saying "no" when someone offers you a cigarette	○	○	○
Saying "no" when someone offers you beer	○	○	○
Saying "no" when someone offers you hard liquor	○	○	○
Saying "no" when someone offers you marijuana	○	○	○
Telling someone they gave you the wrong change	○	○	○
Taking back a product that doesn't work	○	○	○

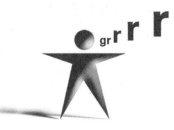

grrr

Coping
with
Anger

Staying in Control

The Warning Light

1. Picture a light inside your head. Imagine that it flashes a warning when you need to stop and think before speaking or acting.

2. Remember to check your light whenever you are in a situation that is making you angry.

Counting to Ten (or Higher)

1. Take a deep breath and start counting slowly to yourself

2. Keep listening to the other person as you count. Don't provoke him or her by revealing what you are doing.

3. Look the other person in the eye.

Self-Statements

Sometimes just telling yourself not to get angry can help keep you calm. Examples of effective self-statements:

- I don't have to let this get to me.

- I don't need to fight about this.

- I can handle this.

- I can stay calm.

- I enjoy feeling calm and in control.

Reframe

Get a picture of the situation that's making you angry. Then put a different frame on it. Ask yourself questions like these:

- Is this worth getting angry about?

- Am I sure this person is really out to hurt or insult me?

- Is there another way to get what I want?

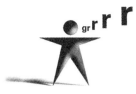

Coping With Anger

Everyone gets annoyed by one thing or another. List and rate the situations that made you angry this week. Be specific.

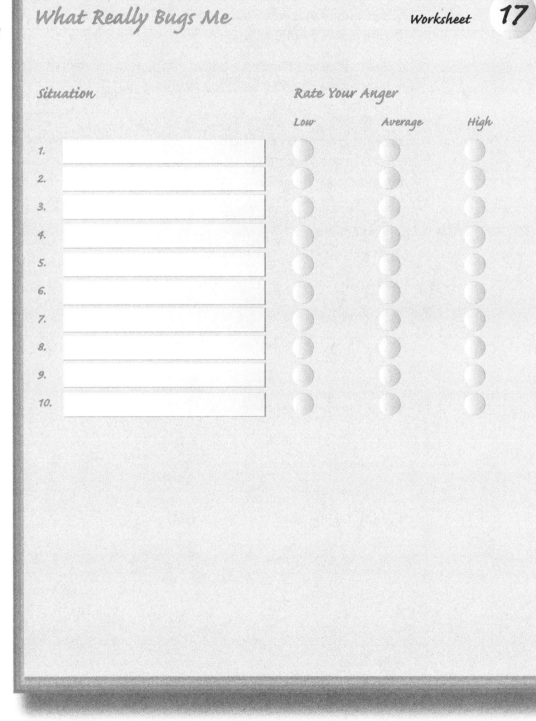

What Really Bugs Me

Situation

Rate Your Anger

	Low	Average	High
1.	○	○	○
2.	○	○	○
3.	○	○	○
4.	○	○	○
5.	○	○	○
6.	○	○	○
7.	○	○	○
8.	○	○	○
9.	○	○	○
10.	○	○	○

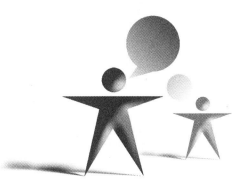

Communication skills

Why Communication Skills are Important

Since we spend most of our lives with other people, it is important to learn how to get along with others. Learning to communicate effectively can help. Communication is the process by which a person sends a message to another person for the purpose of transmitting information or getting a response. Good communication skills can help us develop satisfying and healthy relationships. On the other hand, poor communication skills can get in the way of forming and maintaining satisfying relationships, and can lead to misunderstandings and bad feelings.

Types of Communication

There are two types or channels of communication: verbal and nonverbal. Verbal communication refers to the specific words that we use as well as the tone and loudness of our voice. Nonverbal communication refers to body language, facial expressions, and gestures. Communication can occur using verbal, nonverbal, or both types of communication. Not sending clear messages using verbal and nonverbal channels of communication or sending different verbal and nonverbal messages can create confusion or result in a misunderstanding.

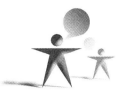

Communication Skills

Looking At Recent Misunderstandings

Describe a recent misunderstanding that you were involved in which resulted from poor communication. (What was the misunderstanding about? Who was the misunderstanding with? How did you feel? How did the other person feel?) Also, identify the specific cause of the misunderstanding and what you or the other person could have done to avoid it.

1. Briefly describe the misunderstanding:

2. What was the cause of the misunderstanding?

3. How could the misunderstanding have been avoided?

Skills for Avoiding Misunderstandings

A misunderstanding is the result of a failure to communicate clearly. The sender communicates one message, but the receiver hears or sees a different one. Below are some simple ways of communicating clearly and avoiding confusing communications or misunderstandings. Practice these skills and use them as often as possible.

1. Send the same message on verbal and non-verbal channels. Make sure what you say and how you say it are the same. Remember, how you say something is often more important than what you say. Your tone of voice, facial expressions, body position, all send important messages. If you say something with the wrong facial expression the person hearing you will be confused. For example, if you say you're mad but smile when you say it, the person you're talking to won't think you are serious.

2. Be specific. Say exactly what you mean. Don't say things in a general way. Unless you are specific, the other person may not know what you mean; they will have to guess. If you say

exactly what you mean they won't have to guess and there won't be room for misunderstandings. For example, instead of saying, "I'll see you Saturday afternoon," give a specific time and place ("I'll come over to your house Saturday at 1 o'clock").

3. Ask questions. This is something that you can do whether you are the person sending a message or receiving it. Asking questions works well if you are telling someone how to do something or explaining something. If someone tells you something that isn't clear, you can ask that person questions as a way of getting more specific information. For example, "I don't understand, can you explain that again?"

4. Paraphrase. Another way of making sure that a message is clear is to use paraphrasing (repeating something back in your own words). If you tell somebody something and you want to make sure they understand, ask them to repeat it back to you. If somebody tells you something and you want to make sure that you understood it correctly, then you can repeat it back to them. For example, after someone has explained something to you, you can say, "Okay, let me make sure I understand what you mean." (Then paraphrase what the person told you.)

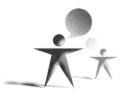

Communication Skills

Read each of the situations to the right and check off the communication skill or skills that could have been used to avoid the misunderstanding or to clearly communicate the message.

Practice Applying Communication Skills

Situation 1

Andrew arranged to meet a friend at the movies on Friday night at seven o'clock. That Friday night, Andrew waited and waited for his friend to show up. He mistakenly concluded that his friend had forgotten or just not bothered to meet him. Meanwhile, his friend was waiting for him at the other movie theatre in town feeling disappointed that Andrew had not shown up or even called to say he wasn't coming.

◯ Send same verbal/non-verbal message   ◯ Be specific

◯ Repeat message back to sender   ◯ Ask questions

Situation 2

Melissa had spent the evening baby-sitting for her new neighbor's three children. It had not gone well. The children had not listened to her, and even locked her out of the house for 15 minutes in the cold! She felt very angry. When her neighbors returned she told them about their children's behavior while smiling and laughing about their antics. The children were promised a trip to the toy store the following day for being so good.

◯ Send same verbal/non-verbal message   ◯ Be specific

◯ Repeat message back to sender   ◯ Ask questions

Situation 3

It was an important field hockey game for Carol's team. They were not having a good season. Their coach had worked hard to come up with an effective game plan that would give them a chance to win. Right before the game everyone met to receive specific instructions for their playing position. Carol really didn't understand her instructions very well. During the game she totally messed up and her team lost.

◯ Send same verbal/non-verbal message   ◯ Be specific

◯ Repeat message back to sender   ◯ Ask questions

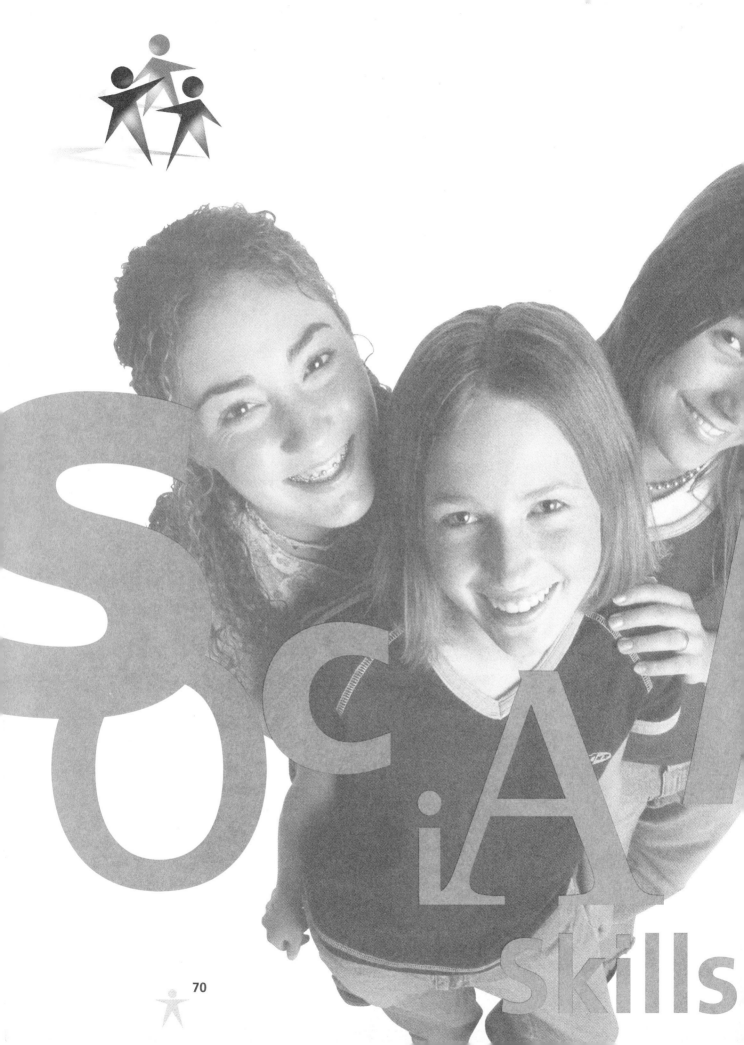

70

Getting Over Being Shy

Many people, even famous TV and movie personalities, can be shy and feel uncomfortable in social situations. However, you can learn to be more comfortable in social situations by learning how to deal with anxiety and nervousness (practiced in the last session) and by improving your social skills in social situations. Below are some ideas.

- **Learn to "act":** You can learn new social skills and become more self-confident by "playing" a social situation as if you were an actor acting out a specific role.

- **Start small:** Begin by practicing on easy situations, gradually working up to more difficult ones.

- **Prepare yourself:** Write out a brief script and rehearse it at home, watch yourself in the mirror and listen to your voice. This is what actors in plays and movies do.

Saying Hello

Another way to get over being shy is to practice saying hello to people. Below are some common greetings.

- "Hello" or "Hi"

- "How is it going?"

- "Good to see you."

- "Have a good (nice) day."

- Gestures (a nod, smile or wave)

    Get in the habit of saying hello to people. The more people you say hello to, the more people who will say hello to you. Most people are shy. You can help them by saying hello first.

"Is that a good book?

Meeting New People

Try to meet a lot of new people. Begin a conversation wherever you go (for example, while standing in line at the movies, grocery store, bank, at a sporting event, etc.). Start the conversation with something you have in common. Again, asking questions is an effective method. Below are some examples.

- "This line is so long, this must be a good movie. Have you heard anything about it?"

- "Is that a good book? What's it about?"

- "That's a nice jacket. Where did you get it?"

- "Did you see the game last night? Who won?"

Giving Compliments

An easy way to start conversations and help others feel good is to give a compliment. You can compliment people by looking at:

- What they are wearing (e.g., "I like your shirt.")

- How they look (e.g., "Your hair looks great.")

- Something they do well (e.g., "You're really good at sports.")

- Their personality (e.g., "You've got a good sense of humor.")

- Other personal features (e.g., "You've got a nice smile.")

Tips for Starting a Conversation

Here are some ideas for starting a conversation with someone you don't know, for example, at a party or dance.

- Pick someone who looks like they would be easy to talk to (a person who seems friendly, is smiling at you, sitting alone or just walking around).

- Introduce yourself. "Hello (Hi), my name is...." Tell each other where you live, go to school, what activities you like (e.g., hobbies, sports, etc.).

- Give a compliment and then ask a question. "You were great in the school play. Do you take acting lessons?"

- Ask for or offer help (e.g., help with a package, lending books or pencils, directions, etc.).

- If you are at a total loss you can use such common but very good starters concerning the weather ("The weather has really been great lately") or personal identity ("Are you from around here?" or "Where do you go to school?")

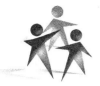 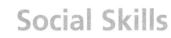

Social Skills

Keeping a Conversation Going

Once you begin a conversation, there are several things that you can do to keep things going.

1. Ask questions.

2. Tell a story about yourself.

3. Get the other person talking about him or herself.

4. Let the other person know you are interested in what they are saying.

5. Be happy and "up."

6. Be an active listener. Show that you are listening by using:

- Verbal cues ("yes," "uh huh," "I see," "that's really interesting").

- Nonverbal cues (leaning forward, standing closer, sitting up, nodding your head, using eye contact).

Ending a Conversation

How you end a conversation can make your next meeting with that person either easier or harder.

1. The ending should be as smooth and natural as possible.

2. Don't cut the other person off in the middle of a sentence. Try to find a natural place to stop.

3. Nonverbal cues can be used to indicate that you want to end the conversation such as breaking eye contact, moving toward the exit, smiling, shaking hands, etc.

4. Be sure the person knows:

- You are about to leave (end the conversation).

- You've enjoyed the conversation (or being with the other person).

- You hope that you will meet (or see each other) again soon.

Use the space on this page to develop social skills "scripts" for giving compliments, starting conversations, and keeping them going. Write down what you could say when giving four compliments, four ways of starting a conversation, and four things you could talk about. This will give you practice with these skills and help you plan what to say in situations involving giving compliments and having conversations.

Developing Social Skills Scripts

Compliments

1.
2.
3.
4.

Conversation Starters

1.
2.
3.
4.

Keeping Conversations Going: Things to Talk About

1.
2.
3.
4.

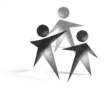

Social Skills

1. Describe the kind of person who you would want as a friend, whom you would want to hang out with.

2. List some social activities that you think might be fun to do with others.

3. Describe an approach that you think might work when you're asking someone out on a date.

Assertiveness

How to be More Assertive

Saying "No"

1. State your position. Tell the other person how you feel about something or give your answer to a request that you do something (e.g., "No, you can't borrow my book.").

2. State your reason. Tell the other person the reason for your position, request, or feelings (e.g., "I'll need to use it myself," or "I already promised that someone else could use it.").

3. Be understanding. Let the other person know that you understood his side, request, or feelings (e.g., "I know you really need to use it, and I wish there was something I could do to help.").

Asking Favors or Asserting Rights

1. State the problem or situation to be changed. Tell the other person what the situation is that needs to be changed.

2. Tell how you might change the situation or solve the problem. Tell the other person what you would like them to do or what you think (asserting rights), or ask for a favor.

How to Say It

Following these tips will help you be more assertive by using the right nonverbal skills.

1. **Loudness of Voice:** Don't whisper or mumble. Speak with a strong, confident tone of voice.

2. **Eye Contact:** Don't look away from the person you are talking to or down at the floor; look directly into his or her eyes.

3. **Facial Expression:** Be certain that your facial expressions are saying what you are saying (for example, don't smile while you are telling someone you're angry).

4. **Distance:** Keep the right distance from the person you are talking with (for example, stand further away if you're telling someone that you've got to go, or stand closer if you're feeling warm or affectionate).

Assertiveness

Some people have difficulty saying what they feel or find it hard to stand up for their rights.

Handling Difficult Situations

1. Describe one common situation where you had this problem with your friends.

2. List the reason(s) why you didn't stand up for your rights or express your true feelings to your friends.

Teenagers are sometimes pressured to smoke cigarettes by their friends or classmates.
1. Describe a situation where you felt pressured to smoke a cigarette.

2. Describe how you handled the situation

Ways of Saying "No"

Simple No: "No." or "No, thanks."

Tell It Like It Is: "No, thanks. I don't smoke."

Give An Excuse: "No, thanks. I'm in a hurry right now. I've got to go."

The Big Stall: "No, thanks. Maybe later."

Changing The Subject: Say no and start talking about something else.

"No, thanks. Hey, did you see the game last night?"

Broken Record: Repeat "no" over and over, or variations on your no response.

"No, thanks."

"No."

"No. I'm not interested."

Walk Away: Say "no" and walk away.

The Cold Shoulder: Ignore the other person.

Avoiding The Situation: Stay away from any situation where you are likely to be pressured to smoke.

Assertiveness

Assertive Action Plan

Here are some common situations that teenagers find themselves in. How would you handle them? What would you say or do?

Situation

You are standing on a long lunch line. Someone cuts ahead of you in line.

You are in a public place where smoking is not allowed. The person next to you lights up a cigarette.

You are in a friend's house and everyone is drinking beer. Your friends ask you to drink. You don't want to.

Your friend wants to borrow your MP3 player from you. You don't want to lend it to your friend since you're afraid it would get broken.

You're at a party where marijuana is being smoked. You do not want to smoke. Someone passes you a joint.

Additional Action Plan

Describe situations that you think you may have to deal with by being assertive. Write down how you plan to handle them.

1. Situation:

Your Response:

2. Situation:

Your Response:

3. Situation:

Your Response:

4. Situation:

Your Response:

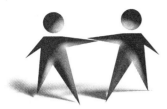

Resolving Conflicts

Changing You and Me to We

1. Stay Cool

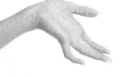

- Take a deep breath.

- Count to ten (or twenty).

- Tell yourself, I'm too cool to get angry.

  I feel good when I stay in control.

  I don't need to fight.

2. Cool Off Your Opponent

- Say: "This isn't worth fighting over."

  Say, "I have nothing against you, and I don't want to fight."

  If someone insults you, ask: "Why would you want to say that?"

- Use your sense of humor to help your opponent lighten up.

3. Listen to the Other Person

- Look him or her in the eye, nod, say "I see."

- Restate what is said, then ask, "Is that right?"

- Don't get too close to the other person. Keep your tone of voice even.

4. Stand Up for Yourself

- Use "I" statements to state your position and tell how you think and feel.

- Give reason for why you feel as you do.

- Stand tall.

- Speak with confidence.

5. Show Respect

- Don't say what's wrong with the other person.

- Say, "I see where you're coming from."

  Say, "I understand why you might feel that way."

- Agree where you can.

- If you've done something wrong, apologize.

6. Solve the Problem

- Suggest a compromise.

- Ask the other person to suggest a compromise.

- Consider other possible solutions.

- Ask problem-solving questions: Why? Why not? What if?

- Consider the possible consequences of each.